HOW TO LOSE WEIGHT AND NEVER FIND IT AGAIN

Danny Crawford

Diligence Publishing Company
Bloomfield, New Jersey

HOW TO LOSE WEIGHT AND NEVER FIND IT AGAIN

To contact the author to speak at your organization, seminar, or conference email: dcrawford691@gmail.com

HOW TO LOSE WEIGHT AND NEVER FIND IT AGAIN

ISBN: 978-1-7374840-5-9

Printed in the United States

DEDICATION

I dedicate this book to my mom and stepfather in heaven. Losing you two was the hardest I have ever been hit. I turned the tragedy into triumph and the loss into a lesson. I will continue to strive to make you proud. Also, I dedicate this book to my three sons Danny III, Deandre, and Devin. Anything and everything is possible. Strive for greatness and never give up.

TABLE OF CONTENTS

ACKNOWLEDGEMENTS AND SPECIAL THANKS

The publishing of this book would not have come to reality if it were not for these people who believed in me and my vision. Special thanks to Aija Tingling, Anissia Barrow, Andre Rodriguez, Antione Crawford, Arlene Jimenez, Aiyisha Shorte, Bradley Hecker, Cynthia Benitez, Charisse Kitt, Derek Huie, Dana George, Dawn and Sean Mickell, Darryl McKnight, Denny Pulido, Eric Reyes, Isaiah Tolbert, Jared Paioff, Jada Eaddy, Jay Reid, Jaime Tibbs, Kanika Williams, Kimberly Thomas, Lina Liu, Laura (YellowShoeLaces) Collins, Lilian Quirindongo, Lashawn Hunter, Lauren Guerrera, Melinda Durgaprasad, Monique Barrow, Margie Ramos-Ciancio, Marisa Diaz, Nicole Garland, Nicole Leary, Roylena Watson-Reynolds, Rashawn Cobourne, Robert Clampet, Steve Rosa, Satonya Wilson, Sherman Blanks, Taena Diaz, Toussaint Tolbert, Thomas Murray, Taniqua Mickell, Thomas Militello, Trina Adams, Tamika Rose, Vanessa Miller, Will Maceo, and Will Santos.

I would also like to give a special thanks to every client that I have trained throughout the years. I learned from you just as much as you learned from me. Thank you for entrusting me with your fitness journey. Some names that stick out: Sheena Chello, Amy White, Sixta Colon (Day ones), Stefanie Johnson, Julie Guadalupe, Star Jenkins, Monique Jordan, Anita Gadsden, Jackie Glass, Tamara Jones, Bonnie Piccirillo, Maribel Havens, Erika George-Riddle, Kathy Jones, Deidre Smith, Richard Minor, Laura Jenson, Karen Perlman and so many more. If I did not mention your name, blame the head not the heart.

I must also thank my loved ones. The ones who I go to for guidance, love, and support. Timara Brown, the Peace you bring to my life is greatly appreciated. You are a blessing. My brother Noel Johnson and sister Makeba Crawford, thank you for being the best siblings any man can ask for. We may not speak every day, but the love is unconditional. My nieces and nephews Troy, Dasia, Vinessa, and Noel Jr. I Love the young men and women you are becoming. Judge Milton Tingling, thank you for being a mentor and always pointing me in the right direction. Judge Marcy Friedman, thank you for always listening to my dreams and encouraging me to go for it. "Aunt "Tinnie" when mommy passed away you stepped in and filled that void. I am forever grateful. My brother Chris Feliciano, 25 years of friendship and the loyalty we have for each other is priceless. My siblings at work Andrew McKiver, Gil Burgos, Xavier Agosto, Floyd Mcgruder, Felix Feliciano, Sherman Blanks, Cecily Hernandez, Kimberly Moses, Saki Bernier, Megan Whitlow, and Melissa Barquinero. We laugh together. We cry together. We are family.

My boy Wax, the respect was there from day one. I'm honored to watch you grow as a businessman and family man. Charisse Kitt, my big sister. I truly am blessed to have you in my corner. You bring so much value to my life. My cousin Magic, you were my very first friend and at the age of 5, you taught me how to read. Now look, I am out here writing books. My cousin Brok, we been through real life battles together and remained solid. Thank you for never filtering your advice and perspective. Your honesty is necessary. Last but certainly not least, I give all praises to God. He saved me on so many occasions. He protected me, guided me, carried me, and taught me lessons no one else could. Thank you.

FOREWORD

From the first time I met Danny back in 2007, I knew he was destined for something greater than who he was. He had all the qualities of someone who wanted more — and every story anyone can tell about him now shows that constant evolution. So, like anyone on a journey, especially in fitness, Danny did not start out with an easy road ahead of him. He struggled, as we all do, but he had one constant that drove him to be a better version of himself — his family. Whether it was the passing of his mother, or the birth of his kids, the internal will to do, and be healthier and successful, at its foundation, can be attributed to them. But he always embodied the image of success with class, charisma, and most importantly, genuineness. Today, as I write this foreword to his first of many published books, I share words that I always hoped — and in many ways knew — I would have the chance to share in dedication to him.

Danny discovered his passion for fitness many years ago when he saw that he needed to make a change in himself. I think that is what makes him able to empathize with those who have weight-loss goals. He tells this story of us back in the academy, when we would be on our run and come back and help those who were struggling to get through, so it is true when they say, "You never know who is watching you, so put your best self forward always."

Over time, he became the one I looked up to for motivation. He would become my friend, my brother, and my trainer. I would always try to be an encourager or give him an encouraging word whether it was through talking to him about his courses for his certifications, listening to his plans to expand on his accreditation and grow his business and platform, or buying merchandise and promoting it in true support of my brother's dreams as he strived to grow into the man we know now. Danny never stops pushing himself, and it is infectious because he will push those around him to be better as well.

Recently, I submitted him for recognition, during Black History Month, for his work in service to the job as an officer, where he has made it his mission to transform himself both mentally and physically to a better person, in health and life, by managing to push himself to achieve his own personal health goals, as well as others on and off the job: from other officers seeking to lose weight, to those wanting to become members of specialized task forces, persons looking to be academy instructors, judges, and other court staff. He has become certified as a personal trainer and built it into a brand that includes not only physical training, but also dietary management and the mental aspects of a healthy life that you can find him speaking about on his podcast. Because of all this work he puts back into the job on his personal time and offers to the community as well, he is considered an authority to go through concerning all things fitness.

It is without a doubt true that fitness has saved his life, but it also has saved others along his journey. And with this book, he will surely help to save more. I am forever proud of the young man I knew back then, and continuously proud of the one I see before me today. May you always be an inspiration to others, and never stop believing in yourself.

Fraternally, Your Brother
Sherman D. Blanks

INTRODUCTION

Overweight and obesity is a serious chronic disease, and the acceptance of obesity continues to rise in the United States. The CDC website reports that this epidemic has been the number one cause of chronic diseases such as high blood pressure, diabetes, heart disease, and cancer. Obesity is often associated with emotional issues such as anxiety, sadness, low self-esteem, and depression. One 2010 study found that people who were obese had a 55 percent greater risk for developing depression over the course of their life than people who were not obese.

I can relate from personal experience of the bad decisions I was making, and my health was taking a direct hit. The moment I decided to live a healthier lifestyle, every area in my life improved. My finances were better. I looked and felt more alive. I was more involved as a parent. I attracted like-minded people that brought value to my life.

I have helped countless men and woman lose weight over the years. However, one problem I came across was I noticed some of my clients would gain the weight back months later after our training sessions were over. Although I was getting results while they were with me, the real success is taking the training wheels off and watching them ride without me. I had begun to question my training methods and decided to change my approach. I researched, studied, and took courses on how to instill behavioral change in my clients. We are all creatures of habit, and most habits are hard to break; especially if you have been conditioned to live and eat a certain way from childhood. I wrote this book to guide you to break down those barriers.

This book will give you the tools and steps to overcome distractions and barriers. You will learn how to work on time management. You will also learn that health and fitness is not an all or nothing way of living. You will have good days and bad days, but it will not discourage you. You will do more good than bad and be intentional on living a healthy life. I can guarantee if you read this book and apply it, you will not only lose weight, but you will also NEVER FIND IT AGAIN. The first step is to turn the page and dive into Chapter One. Let the journey begin.

CHAPTER 1

Set Realistic Goals

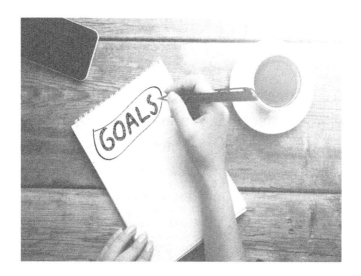

As a personal trainer, I have come across many men and woman with fitness goals that are achievable, but the time they give themselves to complete these goals are unrealistic. There is nothing wrong with aiming high and shooting for the stars. In fact, I encourage that way of thinking. However, when you aim high, you must give yourself the time to get there. You must strategically plan and anticipate distractions and setbacks. If you plan on running a mile in 10 minutes, you must first understand the consistent pace needed to achieve that goal. Or what if you plan a trip from Manhattan to Connecticut by car? The normal time may be one hour, but did you take traffic into consideration? Did you check the GPS to see if there was construction or an accident on your route?

The same mindset applies to setting a fitness goal. You must understand that life happens and along with it comes setbacks. There will always be something that will take you off your journey, force you to stop, slow down, or even take another route. Give yourself that time mentally. This way, if you are aware of the possible bumps in the road, you will not stress and give up. You will keep moving forward until you reach your destination. You may even discover a new path and a new way to get there.

Here is an example of mentally setting realistic goals. I had a client who was close to 250 pounds. When we sat down and discussed her goals, she showed me a picture of a famous Instagram model and said, "I want to look like this by the summer."

I looked at the picture, looked at my client, looked at the picture and looked at my client one more time. The model looked about 5'5" and no more than 135 pounds of muscle, curves, and booty. "Listen," I said to her calmly, "Do you know this person personally? Do you know her story? I'm not trying to take anything from her, but it's 2018 and this can all be manufactured by Dr. Miami or a quick trip to the Dominican Republic."

We shared a little laugh because unfortunately, this is the new way of life. Surgery is the new fitness. But then I got serious with her and said, "Now let us say in fact her body is all natural. Let us say she worked her butt off to achieve this body. There are a lot of men and women that do, and they do not take any short cuts. I promise you it did not take weeks or months. It took years. Years of trial and error, learning what worked for their bodies, failures, mistakes, setbacks, victories, wins, losses, smiles, and even tears. Results like this come from consistency and dedication. Are you willing to dedicate years into achieving that body?"

She looked at me with discouragement and before she could answer, I grabbed her by the hand and said, "The time is going to pass anyway, so how about we aim for it together? Let us make that the goal. In the meantime, between time we will chip away at it and set smaller goals that will get us one step closer. We will enjoy the process and celebrate the small victories we will achieve. It is the first week of November, so let us lose 15 pounds by January. Can we do that?"

She looked at me, smiled and nodded her head and said, "Yes, I think I can do that."

I can tell that by making her mindset realistic and putting it into perspective, she was relieved. She no longer looked at that Instagram model as her body goal. Her goal was to lose those 15 pounds by January, and she believed in herself to do just that. She had begun to set a realistic and achievable goal with the confidence in her eyes needed to make her goal a reality.

S.M.A.R.T.

In the health and fitness world, we use a term called S.M.A.R.T. Goals. S.M.A.R.T. is an acronym that stands for **specific, measurable, attainable, relevant,** and **timely.** When you follow this strategic way of setting goals, you are giving your goals a vision. You are giving your goal or yourself detailed direction that will guide you the entire way. Let us start with the first one.

SPECIFIC: You want to be as specific as possible when coming up with your goal. Let us say your goal is to become healthier. Saying I want to become healthier is too vague, instead you want to say something like, "I want to lose some weight." Now we have a specific goal that we want to reach.

MEASURABLE: This means that you want to be able to calculate your goal in real numbers and details. So, your specific goal is to lose weight. You want to reframe the goal to make it measurable by simply saying, "I want to lose 25 pounds."

ATTAINABLE: Like I said earlier in the text, I encourage you to aim high and shoot for the stars; however, when it comes to your goals, you do not want to aim too high. You want to start small and see early victories. These wins will keep your mind encouraged and motivated. Plus losing 25 pounds in 90 days sounds better than losing

100 pounds in a year. Both are achievable but breaking it down into small goals makes it easier to stick to it.

RELEVANT: This one is the one that is going to keep you motivated. Saying I want to lose 25 pounds in 90 days just is not enough for some people. You need to ask yourself, "Why do I want to lose this weight?" You need something that is relevant to your life. Something that will keep you going even when you do not feel like it. Let us say you are doing all of this because your doctor told you that you are pre-diabetic, and you need to lose the weight to avoid getting diabetes. I do not know about you, but that alone would keep me focused on my goal.

TIMELY: You always want to give yourself a deadline. There is a reason why schools are designed to give students deadlines on projects and assignments. If these strict deadlines were not put in place, nothing would get done. In addition, you want to be calculating when you give yourself a deadline. You do not want to say, "I give myself 6 months to lose 10 pounds." That is way too much time, and you may feel you have plenty of time and will not have a sense of urgency. On the other hand, you do not want to give yourself too little time. This will cause stress, and you may give up because you feel you will not be able to reach your goal in time. I heard a quote by Lisa Nichols. She said, "Your goal is supposed to stretch you, not stress you." This quote is a fact. You want to give yourself a time frame that is challenging but not overwhelming. That will keep you consistent without running around frantically trying to get there and becoming counterproductive. So, let us say for example, you give yourself 90 days. Now you have your S.M.A.R.T. goal. Let us put it together. "I want to lose 25 pounds to avoid diabetes in 90 days." It is specific, measurable, attainable, relevant, and timely. If you apply this strategy, you are guaranteed to reach your goals.

Now that we have discussed the S.M.A.R.T goal, let us move on to some characteristics needed to successfully achieve your goal. One particularly important characteristic needed is the ability to **stay focused**.

When you set a goal, it is inevitable that you will encounter some distractions. Some of these distractions may be devastating. I have been a personal trainer for several years, and I have come across hundreds of clients. Each of them with different personalities, issues, and walks of life. As a trainer you are not just a person that instructs your clients to run, lift, or jump. You become a life coach and a motivator. You become that go to person to help them overcome obstacles. – Not just in the gym, but in life. A good trainer understands that life outside the gym has a way of affecting life inside the gym. So, I encourage my clients to talk to me freely about whatever is bothering them so we can find a solution or figure out a way to get past it, whether it is related to sicknesses, accidents, or even a death in the family. I try to show my clients that there is a way through tragedy to slowly work our way back to taking care of ourselves. I will dig deeper into this in a later chapter.

Although distractions exist, not all are bad, and some are actually a great way to test our discipline, sacrifice, and focus. A prime example of this type of distraction which gets everyone jammed up, is the holiday season. I call them the BIG 3's – Thanksgiving, Christmas and New Year's. People use this as the biggest excuse to fall off track and lose everything they may have worked hard for all year around. I have the biggest plate on Thanksgiving, and there is no way I am turning down sweet potato pie. The same goes for Christmas. On New Year's, I am popping champagne and celebrating life just like the rest of the world because what is the harm, right? Technically it is only 3 days, no big deal. Wrong answer! While I may be stuffing my face with my favorite once-a-year food, I am still staying focused, so those 3 days do not rob me of every muscle I built and pound I lost throughout the year.

So, at this point, I am hoping you are asking yourself, *"How do I stay focused?"*

There are 3 major keys to staying focused on your goals. The first key is to **write your goals down**. You probably heard this before, but there is something about writing your goals down. This technique tells your brain, "This is real."

It is something you can see and touch. It is not a dream or a wish. It is as valid and authentic as a contract. Keep it handy and make copies if you need to. I personally keep my goals on my nightstand, and I look at them every day before I walk out my house. It is a daily reminder that I have something that I am working towards. Also, it is always in my face when I go to bed. At night, it gives me the satisfaction that I am one day closer to achieving that goal.

The second key is **remembering why you started**. This key will coincide with the relevance part of your S.M.A.R.T goals. You can never have too many reasons for why you started. It is good to have several reasons because sometimes your initial reason may not be important to you anymore or your passion for it has changed. For instance, what if you plan on taking a vacation to the Bahamas and you wanted to get in shape for those white sandy beaches? You started a workout regimen, but suddenly your job has a major project, and you must cancel your trip. Now your goal is not relevant anymore. Most people stop and go back to living unhealthy lives. At this moment is where one of my favorite quotes apply, "If you stay ready, you'll never have to get ready."

Despite you goals or reason changing from time to time, always have a few reasons to keep you focused and you will always be ready. That way when the next trip comes around, all you will need to do is make sure your bathing suit fits your new body.

The last key to staying focused on your goal is to **tell people**. Being a man of my word is essential to me. When I tell someone I am going to do something, I do it. When you tell your friends and family your goal, they will hold you accountable. Real friends and family will support you, help you, and even remind you if it looks like you are slipping up. On the flip side, be mindful of who you disclose your aspirations to. There are haters right next to you that will try to distract you from your focus. Pay attention to their actions when you tell them good news. Are they happy when you are happy? Are they always giving you the negative side of a situation when you tell them something positive? They come in all forms. Friends, coworkers, spouses, and family too. Just be aware and treat them accordingly.

Another important characteristic needed to achieve your goal is **patience**. We live in a microwave society nowadays. We want results now. We want instant gratification and the more we advance in technology, the worse it gets. I come from an era of cassette tapes. I remember

13

rewinding my favorite album to get to a certain song I wanted to hear. It was a process. Rewind, stop, play. "Wait I went too far." Fast forward, stop, play. "Nope still not there." Fast Forward, stop, play. The millennials of today will never know that struggle. Now, I grab my phone and simply say, "Play Jay Z's song Dead Presidents," (Yes, I still listen to that album) and instantly the song starts playing. Unfortunately, when we are trying to change our bodies naturally, it does not work that way. It still comes down to one pound at a time. We must consciously get into the mindset that it will take some time and accept it.

A few months ago, I was in the gym with a client, and we were on the treadmill talking and warming up. We have been training for about three months, and she expressed to me that she was not seeing any results in her stomach area. I tried to point out all the other progress we were making, but she was not hearing it.

She said, "I just want to get rid of this gut."

"It'll happen. Be patient," I replied calmly.

"When? I have been doing everything you said. I lost a few pounds but not in my belly," she said sounding more frustrated.

"Unfortunately, we can't choose where the body pulls fat from. It just doesn't work that way," I said. "Honestly, the belly has the most fat pockets and usually it's the last thing to go."

She looked at me and rolled her eyes. I smiled and said to her, "How long have you been eating badly and not working out?" I already knew the answer.

She looked up as if she had to think about it and said in a low tone, "A few years."

"So, you expect to see results in a few months over years of an unhealthy lifestyle?"

She did not reply. She just increased the level on the treadmill and started running.

"Be patient," I said to her. "We'll get there. I promise."

Often, I compare achieving goals to the growth of a flower. The first step in growing a flower is planting a seed. That seed is your initial plan on achieving your goal. When you say you are going to lose weight, you are planting a seed in your mind. The next stage in growing a flower is called germination. During this process, the seed is watered, kept in warm temperatures, and exposed to sunlight. You can compare this with the tools you will need to nurture your goal. You must feed

15

it, keep it protected from outside influences, and expose it to positive energy. Do you see the analogy coming together? When I say feed your goal, I mean provide it with the proper nutrients that will support your growth. If your goal is to lose weight, then is it a good idea to live on a fast-food diet?

In addition, you must keep it protected from outside influences. When your seed is planted and covered in soil, it is protected. It is a must that you treat your goal the same way. The gusty wind of your friends will try to pull your seed from underground to go out for a night of partying and drinks. Plant your goal deep and **stay planted!**

Lastly, expose your goal around positive energy and people. Join Facebook weight loss groups or go to group fitness classes and be around people with similar goals and interests. If a gardener practices this process consistently, the flower will emerge. Some flowers take longer to sprout than others. The gardener must be patient and careful not to do anything extreme to sabotage the process. You are the gardener of your goal, and you need to stay on top of it. Watch your flower grow with pride and look in the mirror and say, "I did that."

After you pat yourself on the back, plant another seed. This seed or goal may be different, so your approach may have to change. Different seeds require different needs, but patience is essential for your flower to bloom.

The last characteristic that I think is especially important to have is **willpower**. Success and failure are separated by a very thin line and decided by your choices. We all are creatures of habit, and it takes a lot of self-control to break those habits. Willpower can be increased but it takes time, and you will once again need to tap into your other characteristics to help you succeed. Here are 3 proven ways to develop strong willpower.

1. Develop Small and Impactful Habits

Developing good habits will inevitably strengthen your willpower. Think of something small yet connected to your goal. The theme of this book is to lose weight, so let us use an example that will support that goal. Let us say you live in a 7-story building and your apartment is on the top floor. You may not be able to walk up the seven flights, but how about one flight? I would advise you to take the elevator to the 6th floor and walk the rest of the way no matter what. Do it every day until you unconsciously press 6 for the 6th floor instead of 7. That small change in your habits will increase your willpower. It will assist in building self-control and self-discipline.

2. Plan Ahead

I had a co-worker that thought it was a good idea to bring donuts to the office for everyone every Tuesday. I am not really a huge donut fan, but that sugar is a drug. I found myself indulging in her kind gesture a few times. I would regret it immediately afterwards and kill myself in the gym trying to burn it off later that day. I decided that I was not as strong willed as I thought I was and came up with a plan. I realized the only reason I fell victim to temptation was because I was hungry. If I ate something healthy and filling prior, the donuts would not be so attractive to me. So, the next Tuesday before I went to work, I ate a cup of oatmeal with cinnamon and cranberries. As I walked past the donuts, I no longer had the urge to grab one. I planned ahead and won the battle of fighting temptation.

3. Meditate for 5-7 Minutes a Day

When you meditate, the idea is to block out everything around you and clear your mind. In the beginning, you will notice your mind begin to wander and then you will have to get it back on track. That same conscious effort used to get back on track is the same exact brain function used when you exercise willpower. As you meditate more often, you will find it easier and less frequent that you will have to tap into your willpower. This teaches you how to better control your impulses.

Once you master these 3 characteristics: **Staying Focused, Patience, and Willpower** you are guaranteed to successfully achieve your realistic goals. Every one of these characteristics is designed to support you as you encounter distractions, setbacks, and everything else life throws at you. When you utilize these tools, it is like that Beats by Dre commercial where an NBA player is walking into the stadium. The haters and media are screaming negative comments or asking distracting questions. The NBA player puts his headphones on and blocks out the unnecessary noise and hears only what he wants to hear.

CHAPTER 2

Get In The Game

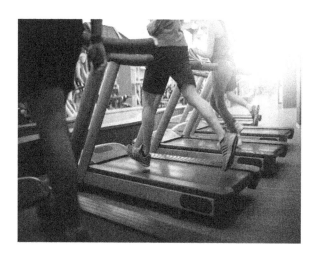

We all know that old phrase "you have to be in it to win it." So, for you to win and fulfill your goals, you must get in the game. When I say get in the game, I mean get a gym membership, join a fitness class, or hire a personal trainer. All of these are investments that will keep you inspired throughout your weight loss journey. Let us explore each one and break down the pros and cons. By doing this it will give you a better understanding of what will work best for you.

GETTING A GYM MEMBERSHIP:

So, it is January the 1st and ever since Thanksgiving that New Year's resolution was on your brain. In the middle of those big turkey dinners and pies, you and your family discussed how you all were going to get fit and lose weight starting in January. In 2017, the global health club industry grossed $87.2 billion with January proving to be one of, if not the most profitable times of the year. Millions of men and women flock to the gym motivated and determined to shed those extra pounds they put on during the holiday season. However, an exceedingly small percentage stick to it and the attendance quickly dwindles down as the weeks pass. Let us explore the pros and cons and maybe we can find the reason.

Pro: Gyms have an abundance of equipment to choose from. From free weights, machines, treadmills, bikes, and ellipticals. This variety of equipment provides everything you will need to start your fitness journey.

Con: No guidance. If you are new to the gym and working out, all this equipment can be quite overwhelming. I can name numerous times I've witnessed gym members walking around aimlessly jumping from machine to machine not knowing what to do. After a while they will get discouraged and stop coming.

Pro: Affordable. There are so many gyms to choose from, you will be sure to find one that fits your budget.

Con: Contracts. A lot of these gyms try to lock you in for an entire year and will charge you a very pricy cancellation fee. Make sure you read the fine print before signing anything.

Pro: Joining a gym can be very motivating. There is something about seeing other people working out and sweating that will make you want to participate.

Con: On the other hand, some people are self-conscious and do not like to be watched while working out.

Pro: You can meet like-minded people and make new friends that will help you stay on track and vice versa.

23

Con: Gyms tend to get very crowded during certain hours. As a result, you end up waiting around to use certain machines, or rush through your routine to allow other people the use of equipment.

As you can see obtaining a gym membership is not beneficial for everyone. It is all up to your personal preference and tolerance. In my experience I found that some people respond better to niche classes like Yoga, Zumba, Boot Camp, Cycling, etc. There are dozens of classes to choose from. Once you find the one for you, it becomes like a family environment. I have heard stories of people finding their soul mate in a boot camp class. One couple even created an entire boot camp themed wedding.

JOIN A FITNESS CLASS:

As I stated in the previous text, a lot of people find fitness classes to be a better route to take on their fitness journey. We all desire to be a part of something and group exercise classes will provide that for you. Let us explore the pros and cons in joining a fitness class.

Pro: Motivation. Being in a room surrounded by like-minded individuals is inspiring. You are all in it together pushing each other, helping each other, and motivating each other to not give up. The instructor will encourage you to depend on one another and hold each other accountable. I always tell my class, "If you see the person next to you slacking, encourage them to dig deep and keep going."

Con: Slip through the cracks. Sometimes classes are so big an instructor will have a hard time seeing everyone. You can easily slip through the cracks and either not perform the exercise correctly or slack on your workout.

Pro: Accountability. When you go to a class on a regular basis, you will begin to develop relationships with the other participants. You will find yourself feeling obligated to go because Lisa said to you, "See you Thursday" or when you miss a class one of the participants will say, "Hey we didn't see you on Tuesday. We missed you." When you have an instructor or classmate showing genuine concern about your well-being, you tend to not want to disappoint them.

Con: Lack of Individual Programming. When you join a class, it is structured for everyone, not just you. If you have a shoulder injury, some of the workouts can make it worse. A good instructor will show modifications, but you may try to push yourself when you see your other classmates doing the workout. I have had clients that had bad knees, and I would instruct them not to do any jumping. As the class goes on, I would catch them doing a jumping exercise because they wanted to push themselves. Days later, they are in pain because they reinjured their knees.

Pro: Affordable. Group fitness classes tend to be more affordable than a personal training session. Instructors can charge less for a group class because of the number of participants. In addition, a lot of gyms offer group classes free for its members. This will save you a lot of money if you are working on a tight budget.

Con: Competitive. Group classes can become highly competitive. If you are new to working out, this can discourage you from the class. It can make you feel rushed or unsuccessful.

When it comes to joining a fitness class, it is all about personal preference. Some people thrive in these environments and some people hate it. I suggest you try it out. In addition, pay close attention to the instructor. A good instructor will make the class fun, exciting, and effective.

HIRE A PERSONAL TRAINER:

Looking for a personal trainer can be a tedious task. As a personal trainer, I can say 85% of my clients come from referrals. Word of mouth is still the greatest form of marketing. So, when you look for a trainer, try asking your family and friends for recommendations. I know a lot of gyms that have personal trainers on staff, and it can be very overwhelming sometimes. When you sign up to a gym, you are immediately approached and offered a "free" assessment. During this assessment, the trainer's job is to get you to purchase a personal training package. Some people feel pressured and sign up without having the opportunity to shop around or even see if the trainer is a good fit for their goals and personality. Being a personal trainer is more than just instructing your clients to pick things up and put them down. A skilled trainer not only trains your body, he or she will train your mind. They will provide you the tools and the mindset to make healthy lifestyle changes that you can utilize outside of the gym. Your personal trainer should be certified by an accredited personal training certificate program. However, just having a certificate does not qualify you as a good trainer. When you meet a trainer, ask them this set of questions: How long have you been training? Do you have before and after pics of your clients? What is your fitness specialty? What is your training style? These questions should help you decide whether they are a good fit for you. Remember this is all about you. You want to be comfortable and motivated. A good trainer will have you looking forward to meeting up with them for a session. Now let us get into the pros and cons of hiring a personal trainer.

Pro: Individualized Attention. When you hire a personal trainer, their job is to focus on you. This is greatly beneficial because they will correct your form, improve your technique, and make the necessary adjustments to your workouts according to your capabilities.

Con: Expensive. Personal trainers can be very pricey. Most trainers will charge no less than $60 an hour and as much as $200. If you meet with them three times a week, that can be $2400 a month.

Pro: Convenient. When you hire a personal trainer, you set the days and hours that work for your schedule. This is extremely important if you have a busy lifestyle. Routine and structure are crucial.

Con: Aggressive Trainer. Some trainers are overly aggressive and tend to use intimidation and drill sergeant tactics to train their clients. This form of training can have a reverse effect on a client and lower their self-esteem and confidence.

Pro: Personalized Program. Your trainer will create a workout program specifically for you and your fitness level. As you get stronger and more fit, they will adjust your workouts accordingly to keep you challenged.

When you hire a personal trainer, make sure they are the right fit. It can be awfully expensive, and most trainers have a no-refund policy. The right trainer will work on developing a trusting relationship with his or her client. They will instill goal setting and will lead by example in helping you achieve your goals.

In conclusion, whether you get a gym membership, join a fitness class, or hire a personal trainer, you are taking a monumental step in your fitness journey. Each of these routes are investments in your life that should be taken seriously. Sometimes making the decision to "get in the game" is all it takes to put you on the path to success.

CHAPTER 3

Surround Yourself With Fitness Minded People

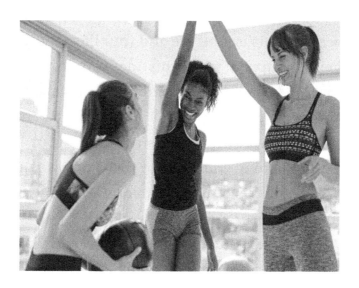

In the words of motivational speaker Jim Rohn, "You are the average of the five people you spend the most time with." The people you spend the most time with shape who you are. If you want to be financially rich, it really will not make sense to hang around broke or unsuccessful people. If you want to be healthy and fit, it would be counterproductive to spend most of your time around friends that frequent fast-food establishments. I know sometimes it is hard to separate yourself from friends or family that have been in your life forever; however, to see change you must change. You cannot keep repeating the same cycle and expect different results. You must remember; this is your life and your life only. They will either support you or distract you. Now, I am not saying to go to the extreme and completely cut them out of your life. All I am saying is think about the role that person is playing in your life. Are they building you up? Are they adding value? Do they hold you accountable? Do their goals align with yours?

When I embarked on my own personal fitness journey, I started to notice some of the people in my life were becoming more distant. I remember Friday nights being the night we would all hang out. We would get drinks, go out to eat and suffer the consequences Saturday morning. However, I started scheduling my workouts for Saturday mornings. Have you ever tried to work out with a hangover? I tried once, and it is the worst feeling in the world. I will never forget hanging out Friday night and I had an 8 a.m. gym session with a client. I rationalized hanging out by saying, "I'll just have my client do all of the workouts. It'll be fine," as I struggled to wake up the next day and practically crawled to the gym.

She noticed immediately. She noticed my energy was off. I am usually enthusiastic and full of life when I meet with my clients. They expect that energy and feed off it. When I opened my mouth to speak, she smelled the alcohol all over my breath and probably seeping from my pores. She said to me, "Wow. Someone had a fun night."

Luckily for me we built a rapport, and she realized I too was human and sometimes make bad decisions. We laughed it off and had a good session. However, I felt very embarrassed and scolded myself for being unprofessional. And to really punish myself, I called her later and told her I would not be charging her for that session and promised it would never happen again. I realized that some of my friends did not align with my goals. They were great friends overall but a huge distraction for where I wanted to be in the next chapters in my life. I had to cut certain ties with them. Some took it personal and would say to me, "You've changed."

To quote the great Jay-Z, "...Like I work this hard to stay the same."

CHAPTER 4

To Drink Or Not To Drink?

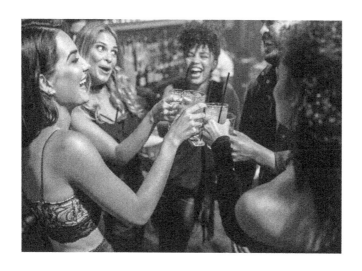

To drink or not to drink? I am dedicating an entire chapter to alcohol because of my personal experiences as well as the overwhelming epidemic of its effect in America and around the world. Since the beginning of time, alcohol has been the number one substance used for celebration. We "toast" to a new job. We "toast" to marriage. We "toast" to new life. We even "toast" to Fridays after a rough week. As a culture, it is just what we do. Now on the other hand, we also go to alcohol to cope with pain, loss, depression, and anxiety. We use alcohol as a means of escape. We use alcohol as a mask. We use it as an excuse to act or say what we really feel. It is a defense mechanism when we hurt someone. It is quite common for us to lash out and apologize later and "blame it on the alcohol."

Growing up, alcohol was a major part of my life. Both of my parents were alcoholics. My mom was what you would call a weekend alcoholic. She would not drink during the week, but Friday nights it was on. After working hard all week, she felt she deserved it. A few years ago, I heard a story about two brothers that lived with two alcoholic parents. They watched as both of their parents would drink every day. They witnessed the negative effects of alcohol their entire childhood. When they became adults, one brother followed in his parent's footsteps and became an alcoholic himself. The other brother never touched alcohol, not one drink. Someone asked the alcoholic brother, "Why do you drink every day?" He said, "I drink every day because I saw my parents drink every day." Then they asked the other brother, "Why don't you drink alcohol?"

The other brother said, "I don't drink because I saw my parents drink every day." They both had the same answer. The moral of the story is life is about choices. Your past experiences should not decide your future. You have the choice and power to change it.

In February of 2008, I received a devastating call that my mother had suddenly died from a massive heart attack. There are not enough words to describe the pain I felt. My mom and I were extremely close, and we spoke every day. It was not long before I turned to alcohol to fill that void of losing my mom. The constant drinking led to rapid weight gain and a decline in my health. This destructive behavior went on for a few years.

In 2012, my fiancé became pregnant with my third child. The birth of my son made me reflect on my life and my health. Do I want to die early and leave my three sons without a father? Do I want them to see me drunk, incoherent, and self-destructing? Do I want them to feel the pain I felt from losing my mom and possibly repeat the same cycle? I decided it was time for a change. I decided to prioritize my health and lead by example for my sons. You hear a lot of people say they will die for their kids. I challenge you to live for them.

How does alcohol affect your weight loss aspirations? I am going to list 3 ways alcohol gets in the way of your weight loss journey.

1. EMPTY CALORIES

Alcohol is often referred to as "empty calories." This means you are taking in lots of calories with little to no nutrients. A 12-ounce can of beer is about 155 calories. A 5-ounce glass of red wine is about 125 calories. So, a weekend of drinking can add up to 1000 empty calories consumed. Also, if you have drinks with soda, mixers, or fruit juice, that contains even more calories.

2. BEER GUT

The "beer gut" is not just a myth. When you consume foods and drinks that are high in simple sugars, they are also high in calories. This will rapidly lead to weight gain. When we work out, we cannot choose where to lose the fat. The same rule applies when we put on fat. Our abdominal area contains the most fat pockets in our bodies. So, when we pack on the pounds, it tends to accumulate in that area.

3. BAD DECISIONS

It is a known fact that alcohol lowers inhibitions and will lead to poor decision making. Alcohol is also known to increase appetite and will have you taking in too many calories. I personally craved pizza every time I would drink. You can easily consume over 2000 calories in one night of eating and drinking. You do that a few times a month, and it is inevitable that you will gain weight.

Do you have to give up alcohol completely? The short answer is no. You can still lose weight and drink occasionally. Some studies suggest that alcohol can have health benefits. It has been scientifically proven that a glass of red wine a day may lower the risk for heart disease. It is the abuse and overuse of alcohol that can have negative consequences in weight management. Moderation is key and cutting back on your alcohol intake will have significant benefits in losing weight.

CHAPTER 5

Learn To Love Your Body

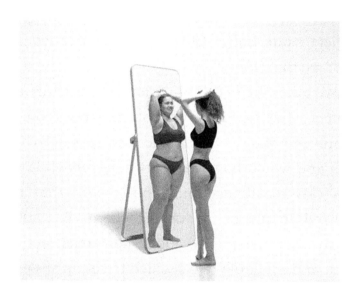

D o you love your body? I would ask my clients
this question often and they would quickly
say they hate or dislike their body or certain areas
of their body. They would say, "I love my legs, but
I hate my stomach." Or "I love my butt, but I hate
my flabby arms." The problem with this way of
thinking and speaking is it's too negative. I am a

firm believer in words being powerful. The things you think or say will manifest into reality. I would follow up that question with another series of questions. "Do you take care of things you hate? Do you respect things you hate or dislike?" When you speak hate or dislike about yourself, you are subconsciously telling yourself to destroy or neglect your body. Change that narrative and start saying, "I love my body."

We take care of things we love. We nurture and protect what we love. Yes, you may see room for improvement, but speak life and love into that area and watch how you start to approach it.

I can recall meeting a new client that was referred to me by a current client. We talked briefly over the phone about her goals, activity level, and schedule. We decided to set up sessions three times a week for 60 days. I knew from our initial conversation that she had some deep-rooted insecurities. She spoke about how she used to look and how much she hates looking at herself now. She has taken all the mirrors down in her house and only posts pictures on social media from the neck up. She was 32 years old and a mother of two highly active toddlers. She stood at 5'4 and weighed about 170 pounds. Her goal weight was 135 pounds. She said this was her pre-pregnancy weight and she would love to get back to that size. I knew as a trainer that I would also have to work on helping her build her confidence. When we met up, I gave her my speech on learning to love your body, but she was so deep into her insecurities she could not imagine loving what she saw in the mirror. I knew it was going to be a challenge to build up her confidence, but for her to stay consistent with the training and reach her weight loss goal it had to be done. I started off by setting small goals during our sessions that were a little challenging for her but doable with the right push and guidance. After accessing her capabilities, strengths, and weaknesses, I was ready to set her first goal. She did not realize it, but she had good upper body strength. I made sure to point that out to her.

"Wow you have really strong arms," I said to her as she curled the 15-pound dumbbells.

"Thank you," she said back with a confident smile.

"How did your arms get so strong?" I asked, really wanting to know.

"Well, my youngest son was so spoiled and never liked to be in his stroller or walk. I literally carried him everywhere," she replied laughing.

Now there it was. I found her strength and I was going to use that as the foundation to every time we came across a challenging obstacle. The next time we met up, I told her we would be increasing the weights to 20 pounds but the same amount of reps. She looked at me like I was crazy, and I could tell she did not think it was possible. As we started the exercise, I noticed towards the end she started to struggle. This is when I tapped into her past experience to help her push through.

"Come on you got... two more. Come on don't drop the baby," I said.

"Ughhh!" she screamed out as she finished her reps.

She was so amazed and felt so accomplished after our session that day. She walked out of the gym just a little more confident than she did walking into the gym. Her head was high. Her shoulders were up, and I even felt a tighter grip when she shook my hand goodbye. After our 60 days, she took the training wheels off and was in the gym consistently chasing more goals. Her last weigh in weight with me was 148 pounds. She is a lot closer to her goal weight, and she is motivated to reach it. She loves her body now, and her self-esteem is amazing. I notice her social media pictures are full body and big smiles. Being a personal trainer is not about barking orders. It is about learning your clients and helping them improve physically and mentally.

Many of us, if not all of us, want to look good on the outside. Let us be real. We go to the gym to look good. And when we look good, we feel good. Being healthy and in good shape is usually secondary in our minds. It is more like a bonus. I too want to look good, but I realized that at a certain age we all start to look the same. Of course, some start to age faster than others, and being unhealthy plays a huge part in aging. However, eventually the wrinkles will come. Gravity will take its course, and things will inevitably begin to sag. So, I no longer focus on the physical attributes more than I focus on living a better quality of life in my senior years.

According to alzheimers.org, "Of all the lifestyle changes that have been studied, taking regular physical exercise appears to be one of the best things that you can do to reduce your risk of getting dementia. Several prospective studies have looked at middle-aged people and the effects of physical exercise on their thinking and memory in later life. Combining the results of 11 studies shows that regular exercise can significantly reduce the risk of developing dementia by about 30 percent. For Alzheimer's disease specifically, the risk was reduced by 45 percent." As a parent, knowing I can be proactive in preventing this disease motivates me even more. The thought of losing my precious memories I share with my children and family frightens me. My great-great grandmother, Irene Crawford, died at 96 years old. I can recall the doctor telling the family how mentally sharp she still was. She was aware of everything going on during her last days. He said, "If her body and organs were as young and strong as her mind, she may have lived another 10 years." Now that is what I call living a long fulfilling life.

Do you know someone in their late 50's or 60's with all types of physical ailments? It is either a bad back, bad knees, hips, etc. Yes, we can suffer from an injury that can cause these issues; however, a lot of times these ailments are from lack of movement and exercise. Have you ever heard of the term "movement is medicine?" When you live an active lifestyle, it will have significant benefits for you in your later years. An active lifestyle will allow you to have stronger bones, muscles and joints and a lower risk of developing osteoporosis. Would you rather be able to run around with your grandkids and relive your youthful days or watch from the sideline wishing you could?

As you can see, loving your body will not only boost your confidence and self-esteem. It will also improve your quality of life in your senior years. Your older self will look in the mirror and see the younger version of you and say thank you. If you take care of your body now, your body will take care of you later.

CHAPTER 6

Mind And Body Connection

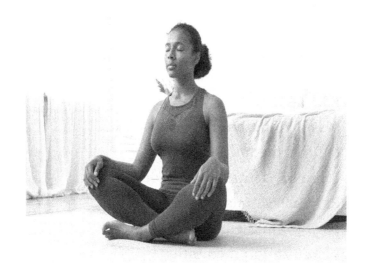

Did you know meditation is an effective approach for weight loss? Let us explore the definition of meditation and how it can help you on your weight loss journey. The Cambridge dictionary defines meditation as "the act of giving your attention to only one thing, either as a religious activity or as a way of becoming calm and relaxed," or "serious thought or study, or the product of this activity." So, meditation can involve breathing exercises, focus, relaxing, and manifesting.

There are nine popular types of meditation practice:

1. Mindfulness meditation
2. Spiritual meditation
3. Focused meditation
4. Movement meditation
5. Mantra meditation
6. Transcendental meditation
7. Progressive relaxation
8. Loving-kindness meditation
9. Visualization meditation

I believe that all these types of meditation can be beneficial in helping you lose weight. However, I find the most effective meditation technique is mindfulness meditation. Mindfulness meditation is a technique that trains you to slow down racing thoughts and let go of negative thoughts. A lot of times we overeat or eat "bad" foods because of stress, anxiety, and worry. Practicing mindfulness meditation will help alleviate those thoughts which will help you make better choices. In addition, mindfulness mediation is the act of being present and paying attention to your senses. Some people have a hard time meditating because they struggle with distracting thoughts or their surroundings. The first thing you want to do when you get prepared to meditate is find a quiet place to sit or lay down. Also set aside at least 5 minutes of no interruptions. Lastly, put yourself in a judgement-free mindset. You may not be able to fully focus the first few times; but remember, meditation is a practice, so it is never perfect. Just keep practicing, and you will inevitably get better at it.

Here are 3 things that will help you during your mindfulness meditation practice. **Notice your thoughts, focus on breathing,** and **regroup.** When I say notice your thoughts, I want you to get comfortable in acknowledging your thoughts. When you are meditating, pay attention to what thoughts come to mind and do not ignore them. Remain calm, control your emotions, and do not let your thoughts rattle you. Do not get caught up in trying to dissect your thinking. Your meditation time is not the time to solve a problem or dwell on an issue. Let the thoughts come and then let them go. The best way to let them go is the second technique, Focus on Breathing. Inhale and exhale effortlessly but intentionally. Feel your stomach rise and fall as the air enters and exits your body. Your body will naturally fall into a calming state. Lastly, Regroup. When you meditate, you will naturally lose focus or begin to over think. Especially in the beginning. You will find yourself feeling worried, fear, anxiety, or stress. It is to be expected and it is okay. Do not beat yourself up about it. Get back to focusing on your breathing. The practice of returning to your breath is the practice of mindfulness.

When you add mindfulness meditation to your daily routine, you will experience benefits physically as well as mentally. The benefits are reduced stress, lower heart rate, improved immunity, and better sleep. All these benefits will play an instrumental role in weight loss and keeping the weight off.

Mindfulness meditation can be intimidating when you are just getting started. I strongly recommend utilizing an app on your phone or finding a YouTube channel that can help. The resources are out there. You can also find books, blogs, websites, and groups that can add great value to your life.

CHAPTER 7

Get Checked Out

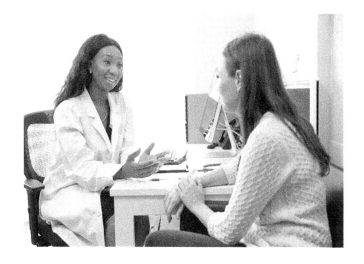

There is a big stereotype about men, especially African American men, that we do not like to go to the doctor. I think it is because every time we go, the doctor tells us something we do not want to hear. I used to be that way, but when I adopted a healthy lifestyle, I no longer had a fear of going to the doctor. I looked forward to it because I knew I was in great shape, and my doctor would give me nothing but good news. However, in July of 2018, I received some shocking and frightening news. I was getting my annual checkup and the doctor decided to give me an EKG. An EKG is an Electrocardiogram. It is a graph of voltage versus time of the electrical activity of the heart using electrodes placed on the skin. My mother died at 49 years old from a massive heart attack, so my Dr. decided to just be on the safe side and check on my heart. Each time your heart beats, an electrical signal travels through the heart. An EKG can show if your heart is beating at a normal rate and strength. It also helps show the size and position of your heart's chambers. An abnormal EKG can be a sign of heart disease or damage. And guess what? My EKG came back abnormal.

"Abnormal? What does that mean?" I asked the doctor trying to sound calm and composed.

"Well, it appears you have some thickening in your heart. I can't tell how thick it is from the EKG. I'll have to refer you to a cardiologist for further testing," he replied.

"But what does thickening of the heart mean?" I asked.

"Well, in some cases thickening of the heart can be a sign of a heart disease called hypertrophic cardiomyopathy."

"Hypo what?"

"It's known to be hereditary. Do you know if your mom had this disease?" he asked.

"No. I never heard of it until now."

"Well, I'm going to refer you to a cardiologist. He will be able to explain it to you in greater detail, and he will also give you an MRI. The appointment will be in two weeks. In the meantime, I do not want you to do anything strenuous. That means no working out."

"No working out? Why?" I asked. Now I was really worried.

"Well, I don't know how thick your heart muscles are, and I just want to be on the safe side," he said.

I did not ask any more questions. I could not wait to get out of there so I could google this disease. That was a bad idea. As soon as I got to my car, I was on Google and YouTube looking up every fact about this disease. I read one story about a college basketball player named Hank Gathers. Hank Gathers played for the Loyola Marymount Lions. He was an amazing athlete well on his way to the NBA. On Sunday, March 4, 1990, the Lions would face Portland. Gathers had just scored an impressive slam dunk. As he was going back on defense, he gave his teammate a high five. Seconds later, he collapsed without warning. He fell so hard the entire gym heard him. He tried to recover but struggled and fell on his back and lost consciousness. He was taken out on a stretcher, and the team physician began cardiopulmonary resuscitation. Gathers was pronounced dead at 6:55 p.m. that evening.

After I read that story, I started going down a rabbit hole of other stories like this one. I read story after story about athletes suddenly dropping dead on the court or on the field. So, this is why my doctor advised me not to do anything strenuous or workout. As a personal trainer, I prided myself as the trainer that worked out with his clients. I used it for marketing. I would always say, "If you sweat, I sweat" or "your goals are my goals."

So while they were on the treadmill running, I was on the one right next to them running with them. If they were doing dumbbell squats, so was I. I would even take it a step further and run at a faster speed or lift a heavier weight to even out the intensity. I literally wanted to feel what they felt, and my clients began expecting that style of training from me. So, when the doctor gave the orders not to work out for two weeks, it took a little energy and motivation from the workout. So, after one week of trying not to work out, I could not take it anymore and started working out again. It probably was not a good idea, but I felt miserable not being able to work out.

A few weeks later, I met up with my cardiologist, and they ran all the necessary tests. They gave me a stress test that felt really weird. A stress test shows how your heart works during physical activity. Exercise makes your heart pump harder and faster; an exercise stress test can reveal problems with blood flow within your heart. So, for them to test you, you as the patient would usually walk or run on a treadmill or ride a stationary bike while your heart rhythm, blood pressure and breathing are closely monitored. However, because I exercise on a regular basis, the doctor felt the exercise stress test would probably take too long. He suggested I take a drug that mimics the effects of exercise. They literally lie you down on a table and inject you with this medicine. Within seconds, it felt like I was running top speed on a treadmill. My results came back normal, so the doctor recommended an MRI. A few days later, the MRI the results came back confirming that I do have thickening in my heart. The good news is its non-obstructive, which means it is not causing any stoppage to my blood flow. However, I must get an MRI twice a year for the rest of my life to make sure it does not get any thicker. It is really a hard pill to swallow knowing I have this condition. I am aware of it, but I refuse to let it stop me from being active and helping my clients. I must admit, I am a lot more careful of my workout intensity and try to monitor my heart rate when I do exercise.

I decided to share this story simply because you just never know. Here I am thinking I am the picture of health, and it turns out I have an underlying heart condition. I also think that if I did not practice a healthy lifestyle, that heart condition would probably be worse right now. Most of the time, one underlying condition has a domino effect. All our organs are connected so if one is not functioning properly, it will cause other organs to work harder to compensate. This will eventually lead to overcompensation, and next thing you know, you will have a whole list of problems and a whole list of medications to treat them.

When it comes to your health, you must be proactive not reactive. I genuinely believe that beautiful people come in all shapes and sizes. And just because you are slim, it does not mean you are healthy. However, you will not see an obese person and say they are healthy. And unfortunately, most obese people live short lives. The sad part is, they die from preventable diseases – high blood pressure, high cholesterol, diabetes, heart disease, and even cancer. These diseases are all due to a sedentary lifestyle and poor eating habits. Let us tackle these two contributing factors.

Sedentary Lifestyle: There are a lot of reasons why we live a sedentary lifestyle. The number one reason is your career. You might be surprised, but 80% of contemporary jobs are sedentary or involve only light activity. Even though you are sitting all day, you do not feel like you are resting because your brain is working. It is like driving a car. I remember I drove to Pennsylvania from New York, and it was a 3-hour trip. Of course, I was sitting the entire time but when I reached my destination, I was so tired. I was tired because my brain did not get to rest. I had to remain alert and focused. It is the same when you are at work; so a lot of times when people get off work, they do not have the energy to go exercise. What is the solution? Go to the gym before work? Yes, that is an option and there are plenty of people that do. However, what if you have kids and you must get them ready for school? So, between taking the kids to school, going to work, coming home to cook, clean, and help with homework, the last thing you want to do is exercise. Trust me, I get it and I can empathize with all those barriers you face.

So instead of being cliché and saying, "If you really want it, you'll make time," or "You have to sacrifice to reach your goals," which I believe is all true, but sometimes the best answer is advising my clients to take small steps. How about we be more active at that desk? Can you ask your boss for a standing desk? Or how about those little exercise machines you can use while sitting at your desk? You will be surprised at how every little bit counts. Set a timer on your phone to get up, stretch, and move every hour. Instead of making your teenage son take the garbage out, pick a few days out of the week and you walk and take the garbage out. And while you are at it, do some walking lunges when you walk back. The moral of the story is you do not have to go to the gym for an hour. The recommendation is to be active for at least 30 minutes a day. It does not say the 30 minutes has to be consecutive. You can break it down into 10-minute intervals.

These are just a few examples to help you live a more active lifestyle. Be creative, research, think outside the box and see what works for you. Lastly, a lunch break is typically one hour. If you bring your lunch, it only takes about 15 to 20 minutes to eat. After that you can go for a nice walk. I am just saying.

Poor Eating Habits: What are poor eating habits? Poor eating habits are when you overly consume foods with little nutritional value that contain high levels of sugar, salt, and carbohydrates. The next question is, why do we eat these foods if we know the effects on our health? There is not just one answer. A lot of times we eat poorly because of our social economic status. For example, I grew up in a poor neighborhood. Money and food were not always available, so we ate whatever we could get our hands on, and the cheaper the food the better because that meant we could get more of it. Most healthy foods cost more, and it was a lot easier to feed your family off the dollar menu in McDonald's than to buy burger meat by the pound in the supermarket. So Chinese food and fast food were always on the menu.

Furthermore, poor people are not the only ones that fall victim to eating unhealthy foods. Close to 46 percent of adults and 56 percent of children in the United States have an overall poor-quality diet. Fast foods are loaded with sugar, salt, grease, and preservatives. And all those ingredients are highly addictive. It has been scientifically proven that when we consume sugar, the tongue's taste buds become activated and send signals to the brain. It causes your feel-good hormones like dopamine to be released. Ironically, the same effect happens when someone sniffs cocaine or heroin. The body then responds by craving more sugar. Chronic consumption numbs the brain's anorexigenic oxytocin system (the sensor that prevents overeating). Basically speaking, your brain does not release hormones to signal that you are full which results in excessive overeating, and we all know what happens after that.

As a wellness coach I recommend that my clients be more conscious of the foods they consume. I know we face many challenges when it comes to our diets. We all come from different backgrounds and cultures, and food has a major role in that. Italians are known for their delicious pasta dishes. African Americans have mastered baked macaroni and cheese and fried chicken. Latinos will add delicious beans and rice to every meal. It is just our culture, and that is how we stay true to our roots.

So how do we honor our culture, eat delicious foods, and eat healthy at the same time? Here is one solution that works for me. It is a word we always hear, and it is called moderation. We must eat in moderation. Too much of anything is not good for you. We can all agree that water is the most important beverage for our bodies. However, you can have too much of it. Yes, you can overdose on water, and it can be potentially life-threatening. Yet to develop water intoxication – or hyponatremia, as it is known medically – you would have to consume an excessive amount of water in a short amount of time. So do not worry too much. Now getting back to eating in moderation. Let me give you an example of what a typical food menu for me would be if my grandmother made me a plate. I am African American, so the meals from my culture consist of baked macaroni and cheese, collard greens, cornbread, fried chicken, ribs, fried fish, black eyed peas, white rice, and candied yams. Not to mention that is just the dinner menu. The breakfast and lunch menus are just as wide ranging. I know some of these meals sound healthy, but grandma is known for adding sugar, salt, and spices for that amazing taste we all love. Also, I am not saying this is all on one plate. I am just giving you a list of the foods that are typically on the menu. If I eat like this occasionally, most likely nothing will happen to me negatively as far as weight gain, hypertension, or any other chronic condition. Chronic diseases and conditions come from chronic behavior and actions. The problem is we eat too much like this and the end results are not good.

The 80/20 Rule
Have you ever heard of the 80/20 rule? Some people use it in relationships, but I like to apply

it to diet and exercise. The 80/20 rule is eating clean, exercising, taking care of your mental health, and minimizing your stress 80% of the time. The 20% is birthday parties, holidays, slip ups, vacations, visiting grandma, and just because you feel like eating ice cream with your kids that day. The truth is if you only indulge in these activities 20% of the time, it will not have a negative effect on your goals.

Keep in mind if you already have a chronic condition such as diabetes, a night of drinking or overindulging on sugar can have a negative effect. So, please be mindful. This is not intended to override your doctor's orders and instructions. This is just a guideline that works for me and the clients that I've personally trained. When I explain the 80/20 rule, people like the idea in theory and it sounds simple enough, but you must really break it down and not just rely on your memory. If you break it down by the week, 20% of 7 days a week is 1.4 days. 80% of 7 days a week is 5.6 days. So, eat clean, exercise, and stay active 5 days a week and indulge a little bit the remaining days. You will lose weight and keep it off. Some people refer to this as the weekend diet. The reason why I support this plan is because it takes the pressure off, and it is not all or nothing. You can still enjoy certain treats, just make sure you earn it and do more good than bad. Lastly, it is not a 50/50 thing. Do not be that person that goes to the fast-food restaurant and order a salad, but then you wash it down with a large sprite and a side of small fries.

In conclusion, like I mentioned in the beginning of the chapter, be proactive and not reactive. Take control of your health and make better choices. Remove the pressure that society and social media puts on you that you must follow a specific way of eating and exercising. The reality is you must do what works for you. This chapter should have helped you understand that you must do more good than bad. You must be active consistently and eat healthy. If you have a seesaw and one side of the seesaw is healthy choices and the other side is unhealthy choices, of course, the one you do more of will tip the seesaw in that direction.

CHAPTER 8

Not So Fast

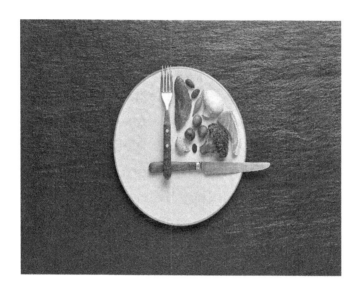

“ Breakfast is the most important meal of the day.” "Milk does a body good." Or how about Dunkin Donuts' genius marketing campaign that convinced us that donuts are a good breakfast choice? Where do these myths come from? Cereal companies played a major role in pushing this narrative that eating breakfast was essential to health. One cereal company that spearheaded this narrative was Kellogg Company. We all should be familiar with the Kellogg's cereal brand. One of the founders, John Harvey Kellogg, was editor of a magazine called Good Health. In 1917, they wrote, "In many ways, BREAKFAST IS THE MOST IMPORTANT MEAL OF THE DAY."

After this article was published, other cereal companies adopted this saying and began to push this phrase with extraordinarily little research to support these claims. Why would they tell us this if it is not true? Well, it is all about getting you to buy into this idea so you can buy their products. I do not believe breakfast is the MOST important meal of the day. I believe every meal is important. I choose not to eat breakfast because of the benefits of fasting. And if you do decide to eat breakfast, do not listen to these ads that try to sell you sugary foods such as pancakes, cereals, and starchy carbohydrates.

Have you ever heard of intermittent fasting? Wikipedia defines intermittent fasting as an umbrella term for various meal timing schedules that cycle between voluntary fasting and non-fasting over a given period. There are a few popular approaches to intermittent fasting.

1. The 16/8 Method

The 16/8 method involves fasting every day for about 16 hours and restricting your daily eating window to 8 hours. I personally practice this method because it is simple to follow. I basically do not eat anything after dinner, and I skip breakfast. My last meal is 8 p.m., and I do not eat until 12 p.m. the next day. Some people wake up hungry and like to eat breakfast, so this can be challenging; so maybe skipping dinner would be easier.

2. The 5:2 Diet

The 5:2 Diet is eating your usual meals 5 days a week and restricting your calorie intake to 500-600 calories 2 days a week. I know a few people that have tried this approach and find it amazingly effective. They find it easier to sacrifice 2 days of low-calorie intake 2 days a week instead of every day.

3. The Warrior Diet

The Warrior Diet was popularized by fitness expert Ori Hofmekler. Typically, you will eat small amounts of fruits and vegetables during the day and eat one big meal at night. If you

71

have a busy schedule during the day and can manage getting through the day off fruits, vegetables, and water, this may work for you. Not to mention, you will appreciate that big meal at the end of the day.

It is important that you eat healthy foods during your eating window. These methods will not be effective if you eat lots of processed foods or an excessive number of calories.

The big question is, what do I do while I am starving, I mean fasting? When I introduce the idea of fasting to my clients the first thing they say is, "I can't do that!" or "I MUST have breakfast in the morning. I won't have energy." I totally agree that food is fuel; however, there are many ways to combat fatigue while fasting. And because of the amazing benefits of fasting, I genuinely believe it is well worth it. Here are a few tips and tricks to boost energy while fasting.

- **Move** – Have you ever dragged yourself into the gym? Your energy was low, and you just did not feel like exercising? But you went anyway. Then suddenly 5 minutes into your workout you feel awake, energized, and motivated. The same effect will happen when fasting. If you just get out and move, your body will respond, and you will get a burst of energy.

- **Hydrate** – When fasting, it is strongly encouraged to drink lots of water. Dehydration causes fatigue. Also, water is an excellent appetite suppressant and can help curb those hunger pangs while fasting.

- **Sleep** – the reason why I choose to skip breakfast when fasting is because it is easier to fast while you are asleep. If I chose the 16:8 method of intermitting fasting, 7-8 of those fasting hours are done while I am sleep. So technically, I am only consciously going without food for 8 hours.

I was training my client Leslie a few years ago, and she was having excellent results. Every week for three months straight, she was losing 2-3 pounds. She was immensely proud of herself and extremely motivated. After the third month, the weight seemed to suddenly stop coming off. She began to feel uninspired and thought her weight loss journey was over. In the fitness world, we call this a plateau. A plateau is a state of little or no change following a period of activity or progress. This happens often and is quite common. There are many ways to break a plateau. One way is to increase your activity level and decrease calorie intake. The program someone uses at 250 pounds to lose weight must change when they go down to 200 pounds. Another effective method to break a plateau is intermittent fasting.

I can recall the day I decided to recommend intermittent fasting to Leslie. We had conversations in the past, and she was a self-proclaimed foodie. She loved going to new restaurants and cooking. She was always in the kitchen trying new recipes from all different cultures. So, I knew telling her to skip a meal was going to be challenging. She had already given me push back when I had her cut calories and portion size on her plates. Now I would be telling her to not eat for 16 hours. I needed more than luck to get her to agree. I needed prayer. Here goes!

"Hey Leslie, have you ever heard of intermittent fasting?" I said while we warmed up on the treadmill.

"Yeah, I heard of it, but I don't know much about it," she replied.

"Well, I know it'll be an effective strategy to help break your plateau," I said.

"Really? What does it entail?" she asked, sounding extremely interested.

I proceeded to tell her all about it, and I noticed she no longer was interested. I knew that may be the case, so I decided to tell her all the great benefits aside from weight loss. As I increased the speed on her treadmill to 4.0 MPH, I started to explain. "There are a lot of changes that occur in your body during fasting. Your blood levels of insulin drop significantly, which opens the door for fat burning. Also, your blood levels of human growth hormone (HGH) will increase. When this happens, your body will begin to burn more fat and help muscle gain. Another great benefit is cellular repair. This process involves removing waste material from cells. Furthermore, it can lower your risk of type 2 diabetes. We all know type 2 diabetes has become an epidemic in recent years. More and more people are becoming diabetic or pre-diabetic. The main cause is high blood sugar levels in the context of insulin resistance. So, by fasting you will reduce

75

insulin resistance, which will lower blood sugar levels and prevent type 2 diabetes."

I can recall Leslie expressing to me that type 2 diabetes ran in her family, and she wanted to break that cycle.

"Wow, all of that?" she asked.

"No there's more," I replied.

We had three more minutes to warm up, so I lowered the speed to 3.5 MPH and increased the incline to 3.0.

"There are several studies that show that intermittent fasting can reduce oxidative stress and inflammation in the body. Oxidative stress is one of the steps towards aging and chronic diseases. Intermittent fasting enhances the body's resistance to oxidative stress. This means it slows down the aging process. Which means you will be the parent that will get confused with being your child's sibling. Additionally, fasting fights against inflammation which causes high blood pressure, arthritis, and other common diseases. So, as you can see, intermittent fasting is a great weight-loss method; but its other benefits extend beyond that. It'll help you look younger, live longer, and fight against chronic diseases that disrupt our quality of life."

"I didn't know not eating for a while would be so beneficial," she said with enthusiasm.

"Yes, I've been doing it myself for years and I never felt better," I bragged.

"Ok let's do it!" she said as she gave me a high five.

A few weeks later, Leslie was all in with intermittent fasting. Of course, in the beginning it took some getting used to, but once she got the hang of it, it became part of her daily routine and lifestyle. One of the benefits I failed to mention was the money she would be saving by skipping a meal. Also, her calorie intake lowered so the weight loss began to happen again. In no time Leslie reached her ideal weight, and now she is in the maintaining phase of her fitness journey. She no longer wants to lose weight, and most of her goals are performance based. For example, she now wants to participate in a half marathon. She still practices intermittent fasting because of all the other amazing benefits. She has even encouraged some of her friends to try it with her.

I have several similar stories from other clients that have adopted the intermittent fasting lifestyle. However, I cannot stress enough to consult with your primary doctor before starting, and once they give you the okay, give it a try.

Lastly, I want to also give you a few cons of intermittent fasting because it is not for everyone.

- ❖ People taking medications that require food
- ❖ Women who are pregnant or trying to conceive
- ❖ Children and teenagers
- ❖ Anyone with a history of disordered eating

These factors can have adverse side effects when you restrict your meals. Just like with any information given, you must do your own independent research and decide based on your personal lifestyle, capabilities, and health.

CHAPTER 9

The Work

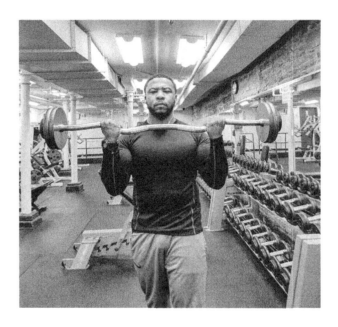

If you made it this far in the book, you may be to the point that you are asking yourself: "So what are the workouts that will help me lose weight?" In this chapter, I intend to give a deep dive into effective workout programs that will aide on your weight-loss journey. When the average person thinks of weight loss, they think of cardio. Cardio is defined as any type of exercise that gets your heart rate up and keeps it up for a prolonged period. That includes but is not limited to running, swimming, elliptical machine use, or bike riding. Cardio exercise has many benefits.

- ❖ Improves Lung Capacity
- ❖ Weight Loss
- ❖ Better Sleep
- ❖ Boosts Immune System
- ❖ Strengthens Your Heart

Those are just a few of the many benefits. I can remember a time when I hated cardio. I hated the uncomfortable feeling I got when I was out of breath. However, I quickly realized the only reason why I hated it so much is because I was out of shape. I started to focus on building up my stamina and endurance. I would set small goals for myself. I would challenge myself to run half a mile without stopping. Then 1 mile, then 2 miles. Soon I was in such great shape I could run 10 miles straight. I know there are some marathon runners out there that run 10 miles with ease, but for me that was a huge milestone. I went from hating to run to being able to run for miles with no problem. I discovered something called the runners high. A runner's high is a feeling of euphoria coupled with reduced anxiety and a lessened ability to feel pain. I have always heard of it but never experienced it personally. When you experience a runner's high, you literally feel like you just conquered the world. So, what does all of this have to do with losing weight? Exercise should not feel like a chore. It should not be something you hate doing.

Initially I can understand the anxiety that comes with starting an exercise program, but the goal is to enjoy and look forward to working out. Cardio is an amazing tool to use on your weight loss journey.

HIIT

One of the most effective training methods that I use is called HIIT. HIIT stands for High Intensity Interval Training. HIIT involves short bursts of intense exercise followed by low-intensity recovery periods. For example, if you were to sprint for 30 seconds and then jog or walk for 2 minutes and do this for a couple of rounds lasting 10-30 minutes, that would be considered a HIIT workout. Here are some of the benefits of adopting a HIIT program.

> ➤ Burn a lot of calories in a short amount of time
> ➤ Fat burning
> ➤ Muscle gain
> ➤ Reduce heart rate and blood pressure
> ➤ Blood sugar can be reduced

There are many ways to add HIIT into your workout routine. Be creative and choose exercises you enjoy and have fun. The best part about HIIT is you can get the same results in 20 minutes that you will get in one hour of traditional workouts. So, if you are short on time, HIIT is the right program for you.

Resistance Training

Now let's get into resistance training. Resistance training or strength training involves the performance of physical exercises which are designed to improve strength and endurance. Most people associate resistance training with lifting weights, but isometrics (planks, wall sits), calisthenics (push-ups, pull ups) and plyometrics (squat jumps, box jumps, clap push-ups) are also a form of resistance training. Resistance training is key to losing weight. When you add resistance training to your program, you will begin to build more lean muscle which means your body will burn more calories at rest. The metabolic demand of a pound of muscle is greater than it is for a pound of fat. This means the more muscles you have, the more calories you burn throughout the day.

Many women are apprehensive to get into strength training because of the misconception that they are going to bulk up and look like a man. Let me be the first to tell you that is far from the truth. The main reason a female cannot gain muscle mass to the same extent as males is the difference in hormone status. The women you see in the media that have that bulky look are chronically using androgenic compounds (steroids) to increase their muscle mass and size. The female that does not go down that route can lift as heavy and as hard as she wants but will never come close to looking like a man. So do not be afraid to pick up those weights and build that strength. Also, strength training will help you perform better when doing cardio exercises. When I would take my clients for a run, and I noticed them struggle I would ask them, "Where do you feel the "pain" – in your lungs or your legs?" If they told me, they felt it in their lungs, I knew we needed to work on their stamina. If they said they felt it in their legs, I knew we needed to work on building the strength in their legs. Sometimes they would say they felt it in their back, which indicates to me that we needed to build up their core strength.

Strength training is what really shapes you. Lifting weights will give you that toned physique, improve your posture, and increase your confidence.

Lastly, do not beat yourself up if you do not see big weight loss results on the scale. I encourage you to take pictures, take your measurements and go by how your clothes fit. Muscle is more compact than fat, and the scale does not know the difference.

When training my clients, we incorporate cardio and strength training to maximize weight loss. If someone only does cardio, they may lose the weight, but they risk losing muscle as well. This will lead to loose skin. To avoid that, you must simultaneously build muscle and burn fat.

If you only do strength training, you miss out on the benefits you gain from cardiovascular exercises. As you can see, cardio and strength training are essential to overall health and fitness and will play a major role in helping you lose weight.

CHAPTER 10

The Journey

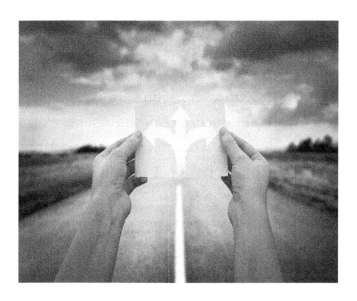

When I first began training clients, my goal was to help them reach their highest fitness potential. I helped them conquer physical abilities they never thought they could – from running their first mile, to competing in body building competitions and coming in first place. Some dreaded our sessions. Others looked forward to it, but all felt empowered after our sessions. I heard a quote a few years ago that said, "If you do what you love, you'll never work another day." That quote could not have been more true. I am forever grateful and honored to be a part of so many people's fitness journey. It is such a rewarding feeling when a client tells me I changed their life for the better. The life we live is indeed a journey. I compare it to being on many road trips with many destinations. As you embark on your journey, you will encounter roadblocks. You will encounter detours. You may even encounter a fender bender. But the goal is to always make it to your destination.

Have you ever been on the highway and noticed everyone slowing down? You would get frustrated when you realize everyone slowed down because they were rubbernecking and looking at an accident on the opposite side of the highway. Then you too look over and slow down as well. Distractions will inevitably happen, and it will slow you down, but do not let it stop you. Furthermore, do not get caught up in one way to reach your destination. There are many roads to your destination, and sometimes the long way is the best way.

In most cases, losing weight can be considered the easy part. The hard part is keeping it off. Keeping the weight off is where the real work begins. It requires more discipline and consistency.

I wrote this book with the intentions of helping you change your mindset when it comes to your health. I challenge you to apply these tools I have provided and use them in your everyday life. Set realistic goals and conquer them. Invest in yourself by getting in the gym or hire a trainer. Learn to love your body because we take care of what we love. Get your mind right by adding meditation to your daily routine. Surround yourself with other health-minded people. Change your eating habits. Go to the doctor often and get checked out. I guarantee you will LOSE WEIGHT AND NEVER FIND IT AGAIN.

ABOUT THE AUTHOR

Danny Crawford is a man of many hats. He is a 14-year Law Enforcement Officer veteran in NYC. He's also the owner and founder of Versatile Fitness LLC where he provides one-on-one training, group training, meal plans, online fitness classes, and wellness coaching. He also hosts a podcast titled "Fitness Saved My Life."

Danny is a Certified Personal Trainer with specializations in Group Personal Training, Weight Loss, and Behavior Change through The National Academy of Sports Medicine. Danny's passion for fitness and helping people led him into the field of personal training and wellness coaching. He's able to relate to his clients because he once struggled with living an unhealthy lifestyle himself.

As a father of three boys, he recognizes the influence he has over them. He strives to guide them in the right direction through his actions and leadership. Danny believes health and fitness is the foundation for success, confidence, and strength.

Hundreds of people have reached out to Danny on a daily basis through social media for advice and tips. This inspired Danny to write his first book "HOW TO LOSE WEIGHT AND NEVER FIND IT AGAIN." This book gives detailed strategies and techniques to not just lose weight but keep it off by changing your way of thinking. Danny uses his personal experiences and his experiences with his clients to deliver a relatable, entertaining, and informative approach to adopting a healthy lifestyle. Whether you're trying to lose weight or trying to maintain the weight you already lost, this is the book for you.

ORDER INFORMATION

You can order additional copies of *How To Lose Weight And Never Find It Again* by emailing the author directly using the email address below.

Danny Crawford

dcrawford691@gmail.com

Books are available at Amazon.com, BN.com Kindle and Your Local Bookstores (By Request)

Please leave a review for this book on Amazon and let other readers know how much you enjoyed reading it.

Thank you!

Made in the USA
Middletown, DE
30 September 2021

48603929R00066